The Keto Vegan Diet
for beginners

Affordable and easy keto vegan recipes for beginners

Susan Muncy

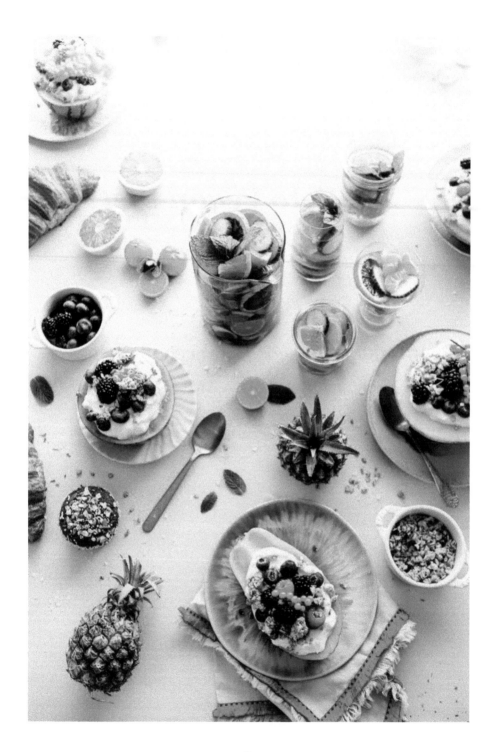

Table of Contents

SOUP

Pesto Pea Soup

Preparation Time: 10 Minutes

Cooking Time: 20 Minutes

Servings: 4

Ingredients:

- 2 cups Water
- 8 oz. Tortellini
- ¼ cup Pesto
- 1 Onion, small & finely chopped
- 1 lb. Peas, frozen
- 1 Carrot, medium & finely chopped
- 1 ¾ cup Vegetable Broth, less sodium
- 1 Celery Rib, medium & finely chopped

Directions:

1. To start with, boil the water in a large pot over a medium-high heat.
2. Next, stir in the tortellini to the pot and cook it following the instructions given in the packet.
3. In the meantime, cook the onion, celery, and carrot in a deep saucepan along with the water and broth.

4. Cook the celery-onion mixture for 6 minutes or until softened.
5. Now, spoon in the peas and allow it to simmer while keeping it uncovered.
6. Cook the peas for few minutes or until they are bright green and soft.
7. Then, spoon in the pesto to the pea's mixture. Combine well.
8. Pour the mixture into a high-speed blender and blend for 2 to 3 minutes or until you get a rich, smooth soup.
9. Return the soup to the pan. Spoon in the cooked tortellini.
10. Finally, pour into a serving bowl and top with more cooked peas if desired.
11. Tip: If desired, you can season it with Maldon salt at the end.

Nutrition: Calories 100 Fat 0 g Protein 0 g Carbohydrates 0 g

Avocado Green Soup

Preparation Time: 5 Minutes

Cooking Time: 5 Minutes

Servings: 4

Ingredients:

- 2 tbsp. olive oil
- 1 ½ cup fresh kale, chopped coarsely
- 1 ½ cup fresh spinach, chopped coarsely
- 3 large avocados, halved, pitted and pulp extracted
- 2 cups of soy milk
- 2 cups no-sodium vegetable broth
- 3 tbsp. chopped fresh mint leaves
- ¼ tsp salt
- ¼ tsp black pepper
- 2 limes, juiced

Directions:

1. Heat the olive oil in a medium saucepan over medium heat and mix in the kale and spinach. Cook until wilted, 3 minutes and turn off the heat.

2. Add the remaining ingredients and using an immersion blender, puree the soup until smooth.

3. Dish the soup and serve immediately.

Nutrition: Calories 400 Fat 10 g Protein 20 g Carbohydrates 30 g

Black Bean Nacho Soup

Preparation Time: 5 Minutes

Cooking Time: 30 Minutes

Servings: 4

Ingredients:

- 30 oz. Black Bean
- 1 tbsp. Olive Oil
- 2 cups Vegetable Stock
- ½ of 1 Onion, large & chopped
- 2 ½ cups Water
- 3 Garlic cloves, minced
- 14 oz. Mild Green Chillies, diced
- 1 tsp. Cumin
- 1 cup Salsa
- ½ tsp. Salt
- 16 oz. Tomato Paste
- ½ tsp. Black Pepper

Directions:

1. For making this delicious fare, heat oil in a large pot over medium-high heat.
2. Once the oil becomes hot, stir in onion and garlic to it.

3. Sauté for 4 minutes or until the onion is softened.

4. Next, spoon in chili powder, salt, cumin, and pepper to the pot. Mix well.

5. Then, stir in tomato paste, salsa, water, green chillies, and vegetable stock to onion mixture. Combine.

6. Bing the mixture to a boil. Allow the veggies to simmer.

7. When the mixture starts simmering, add the beans.

8. Bring the veggie mixture to a simmer again and lower the heat to low.

9. Finally, cook for 15 to 20 minutes and check for seasoning. Add more salt and pepper if needed.

10. Garnish with the topping of your choice. Serve it hot.

Nutrition: Calories 270 Fat 10 g Protein 10 g Carbohydrates 10 g

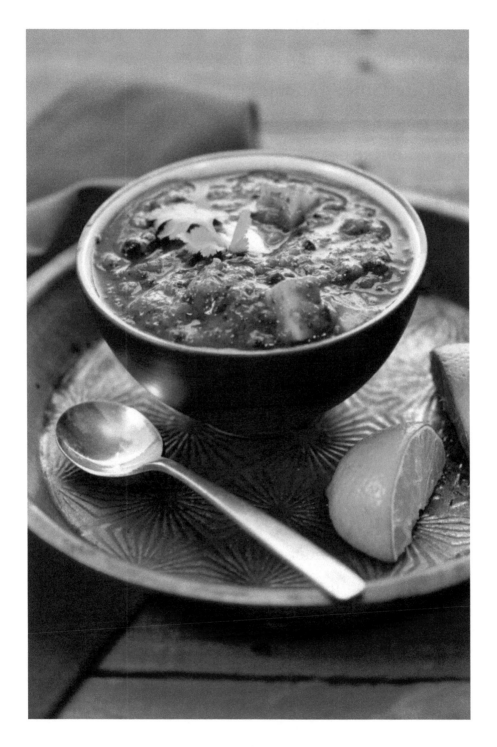

Potato Leek Soup

Preparation Time: 5 Minutes

Cooking Time: 5 Minutes

Servings: 4

Ingredients:

- 1 cup fresh cilantro leaves
- 6 garlic cloves, peeled
- 3 tbsp. vegetable oil
- 3 leeks, white and green parts chopped
- 2 lb. russet potatoes, peeled and chopped
- 1 tsp cumin powder
- ¼ tsp salt
- ¼ tsp black pepper
- 2 bay leaves
- 6 cups no-sodium vegetable broth

Directions:

1. In a spice blender, process the cilantro and garlic until smooth paste forms.
2. Heat the vegetable oil in a large pot and sauté the garlic mixture and leeks until the leeks are tender, 5 minutes.

3. Mix in the remaining ingredients and allow boiling until the potatoes soften, 15 minutes.
4. Turn the heat off, open the lid, remove and discard the bay leaves.
5. Using an immersion blender, puree the soup until smooth.
6. Dish the food and serve warm.

Nutrition: Calories 215 Fat 0 g Protein 10 g Carbohydrates 20.0 g

Lentil Soup

Preparation Time: 15 Minutes

Cooking Time: 25 Minutes

Servings: 4

Ingredients:

- 1 tbsp. Olive Oil
- 4 cups Vegetable Stock
- 1 Onion, finely chopped
- 2 Carrots, medium
- 1 cup Lentils, dried
- 1 tsp. Cumin

Directions:

1. To make this healthy soup, first, you need to heat the oil in a medium-sized skillet over medium heat.
2. Once the oil becomes hot, stir in the cumin and then the onions.
3. Sauté them for 3 minutes or until the onion is slightly transparent and cooked.
4. To this, add the carrots and toss them well.
5. Next, stir in the lentils. Mix well.
6. Now, pour in the vegetable stock and give a good stir until everything comes together.

7. As the soup mixture starts to boil, reduce the heat and allow it to simmer for 10 minutes while keeping the pan covered.
8. Turn off the heat and then transfer the mixture to a bowl.
9. Finally, blend it with an immersion blender or in a high-speed blender for 1 minute or until you get a rich, smooth mixture.
10. Serve it hot and enjoy.

Nutrition: Calories: 266 Fat: 13 Fiber: 8 Carbs: 10 Protein: 11

Kale White Bean Soup

Preparation Time: 10 Minutes

Cooking Time: 45 Minutes

Servings: 4

Ingredients:

- 1 Onion, medium & finely sliced
- 3 cups Kale, coarsely chopped
- 2 tsp. Olive Oil
- 15 oz. White Beans
- 4 cups Vegetable Broth
- 4 Garlic Cloves, minced
- Sea Salt & Pepper, as needed
- 2 tsp. Rosemary, fresh & chopped
- 1 lb. White Potatoes, cubed

Directions:

1. Begin by taking a large saucepan and heat it over a medium-high heat.
2. Once the pan becomes hot, spoon in the oil.
3. Next, stir in the onion and sauté for 8 to 9 minutes or until the onions are cooked and lightly browned.
4. Then, add the garlic and rosemary to the pan.
5. Sauté for a further minute or until aromatic.

6. Now, pour in the broth along with the potatoes, black pepper, and salt. Mix well.

7. Bring the mixture to a boil, and when it starts boiling, lower the heat.

8. Allow it to simmer for 32 to 35 minutes or until the potatoes are cooked and tender.

9. After that, mash the potatoes slightly by using the back of the spoon.

10. Finally, add the kale and beans to the soup and cook for 8 minutes or until the kale is wilted.

11. Check the seasoning. Add more salt and pepper if needed.

12. Serve hot.

Nutrition: Calories: 198 Fat: 11 Fiber: 1 Carbs: 12 Protein: 12

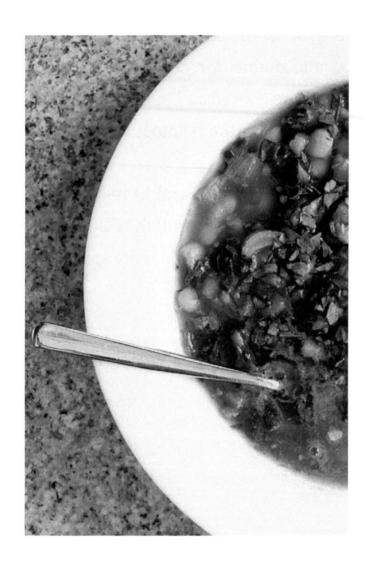

Black Bean Mushroom Soup

Preparation Time: 10 Minutes

Cooking Time: 40 Minutes

Servings: 2

Ingredients:

- 2 tbsp. Olive Oil
- 1 clove of Garlic, peeled & minced
- ½ cup Vegetable Stock
- 1 tsp. Thyme, dried
- 15 oz. Black Beans
- 1 2/3 cup Water, hot
- oz. Mushrooms
- 1 Onion, finely chopped
- 4 Sourdough Bread Slices
- Vegan Butter, to serve

Directions:

1. To begin with, spoon the oil into a medium-sized deep saucepan over a medium heat.
2. Once the oil becomes hot, stir in the onion and garlic.
3. Sauté for 5 minutes or until the onion is translucent.
4. Next, spoon in the mushrooms and thyme. Mix well.

5. Cook for another 5 minutes or until dark brown.

6. Then, pour the water into the mixture along with the stock and beans.

7. Allow it to simmer for 20 minutes or until the mushroom is soft.

8. Pour the mixture to a high-speed blender and pulse for 1 to 2 minutes until it is smooth yet grainy.

9. Serve and enjoy.

Nutrition: Calories: 400 Fat: 32 Fiber: 6 Carbs: 4 Protein: 25

Broccoli Soup

Preparation Time: 5 Minutes

Cooking Time: 15 Minutes

Servings: 2

Ingredients:

- 3 cup Vegetable Broth
- 2 Green Chili
- 2 cups Broccoli Florets
- 1 tbsp. Chia Seeds
- 1 cup Spinach
- 1 tsp. Oil
- 4 Celery Stalk
- 1 Potato, medium & cubed
- 4 Garlic cloves
- Salt, as needed
- Juice of ½ of 1 Lemon

Directions:

1. First, heat the oil in a large sauté pan over a medium-high heat.
2. Once the oil becomes hot, add the potatoes to it.

3. When the potatoes become soft, stir all the remaining ingredients into the pan, excluding the spinach, chia seeds, and lemon.
4. Cook until the broccoli is soft, and then add the spinach and chia seed to the pan.
5. Turn off the heat after cooking for 2 minutes.
6. Allow the spinach mixture to cool slightly. Pour the mixture into a high-speed blender and blend for two minutes or until smooth.
7. Pour the lemon juice over the soup. Stir and serve immediately.
8. Enjoy.

Nutrition: Calories: 200 Fat: 3 Fiber: 2 Carbs: 5 Protein: 4

Mexican Soup

Preparation Time: 10 Minutes

Cooking Time: 45 Minutes

Servings: 6

Ingredients:

- 2 tbsp. Extra Virgin Olive Oil
- 8 oz. can of Diced Tomatoes & Chilies
- 1 Yellow Onion, diced
- 2 cups Green Lentils
- ½ tsp. Salt
- 2 Celery Stalks, diced
- 8 cups Vegetable Broth
- 2 Carrots, peeled & diced
- 2 cups Diced Tomatoes & Juices
- 3 Garlic cloves, minced
- 1 Red Bell Pepper, diced
- 1 tsp. Oregano
- 1 tbsp. Cumin
- ¼ tsp. Smoked Paprika
- 1 Avocado, pitted & diced

Directions:

1. Heat oil in a large-sized pot over a medium heat.

2. Once the oil becomes hot, stir in the onion, bell pepper, carrot, and celery into the pot.
3. Cook the onion mixture for 5 minutes or until the veggies are soft.
4. Then, spoon in garlic, oregano, cumin, and paprika into it and sauté for one minute or until aromatic.
5. Next, add the tomatoes, salt, chilies, broth, and lentils to the mixture.
6. Now, bring the tomato-chili mixture to a boil and allow it to simmer for 32 to 40 minutes or until the lentils become soft.
7. Check the seasoning and add more if needed.
8. Serve along with avocado and hot sauce.

Nutrition: Calories: 344 Fat: 23 Fiber: 12 Carbs: 3 Protein: 16

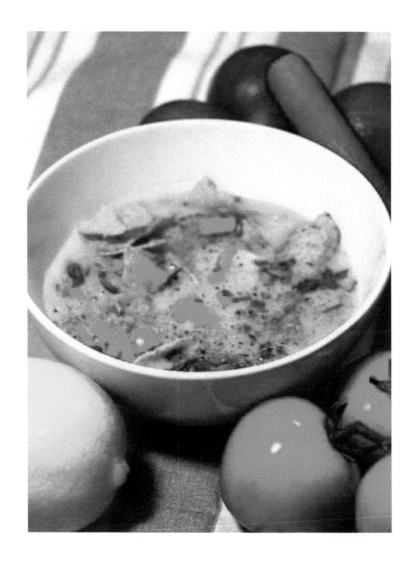

Celery Dill Soup

Preparation Time: 10 Minutes

Cooking Time: 20 Minutes

Servings: 4

Ingredients:

- 2 tbsp. coconut oil
- ½ lb. celery root, trimmed
- 1 garlic clove
- 1 medium white onion
- ¼ cup fresh dill, roughly chopped
- 1 tsp cumin powder
- ¼ tsp nutmeg powder
- 1 small head cauliflower, cut into florets
- 3½ cups seasoned vegetable stock
- 5 oz. vegan butter
- Juice from 1 lemon
- ¼ cup coconut cream
- Salt and black pepper to taste

Directions:

1. Melt the coconut oil in a large pot and sauté the celery root, garlic, and onion until softened and fragrant, 5 minutes.

2. Stir in the dill, cumin, and nutmeg, and stir-fry for 1 minute. Mix in the cauliflower and vegetable stock. Allow the soup to boil for 15 minutes and turn the heat off.
3. Add the vegan butter and lemon juice, and puree the soup using an immersion blender.
4. Stir in the coconut cream, salt, black pepper, and dish the soup.
5. Serve warm.

Nutrition: Calories: 180 Fat: 12 Fiber: 4 Carbs: 5 Protein: 17

Medley of Mushroom Soup

Preparation Time: 10 Minutes

Cooking Time: 20 Minutes

Servings: 4

Ingredients:

- 4 oz. unsalted vegan butter
- 1 small onion, finely chopped
- 1 garlic clove, minced
- 2 cups sliced mixed mushrooms
- ½ lb. celery root, chopped
- ½ tsp dried rosemary
- 3 cups of water
- 1 vegan stock cube, crushed
- 1 tbsp. plain vinegar
- 1 cup coconut cream
- 6 leaves basil, chopped

Directions:

1. Melt the vegan butter in a medium pot and sauté the onion, garlic, mushrooms, celery, and rosemary until the vegetables soften, 5 minutes.

2. Stir in the water, stock cube, and vinegar. Cover the pot, allow boiling, and then, simmer for 10 minutes.

3. Mix in the coconut cream and puree the ingredients using an immersion blender until smooth. Simmer for 2 minutes.

4. Dish the soup and serve warm.

Nutrition: Calories: 140 Fat: 3 Fiber: 2 Carbs: 1. 5 Protein: 7

SMOOTHIES AND BEVERAGES

Kale Smoothie

Preparation Time: 5 minutes

Cooking Time: 0 minutes

Servings: 2

Ingredients:

- 2 cups chopped kale leaves
- 1 banana, peeled
- 1 cup frozen strawberries
- 1 cup unsweetened almond milk
- 4 Medjool dates, pitted and chopped

Directions:

1. Put all the ingredients in a food processor, then blitz until glossy and smooth.
2. Serve immediately or chill in the refrigerator for an hour before serving.

Nutrition: Calories: 663 Fat: 10.0g Carbs: 142.5g Fiber: 19.0g Protein: 17.4g

Hot Tropical Smoothie

Preparation Time: 5 minutes

Cooking Time: 0 minutes

Servings: 4

Ingredients:

- 1 cup frozen mango chunks
- 1 cup frozen pineapple chunks
- 1 small tangerine, peeled and pitted
- 2 cups spinach leaves
- 1 cup coconut water
- ¼ teaspoon cayenne pepper, optional

Directions:

1. Add all the ingredients in a food processor, then blitz until the mixture is smooth and combine well.
2. Serve immediately or chill in the refrigerator for an hour before serving.

Nutrition: Calories: 283 Fat: 1.9g Carbs: 67.9g Fiber: 10.4g Protein: 6.4g

Cranberry and Banana Smoothie

Preparation Time: 5 minutes

Cooking Time: 0 minutes

Servings: 4

Ingredients:

- 1 cup frozen cranberries
- 1 large banana, peeled
- 4 Medjool dates, pitted and chopped
- 1½ cups unsweetened almond milk

Directions:

1. Add all the ingredients in a food processor, then process until the mixture is glossy and well mixed.
2. Serve immediately or chill in the refrigerator for an hour before serving.

Nutrition: Calories: 616 Fat: 8.0g Carbs: 132.8g Fiber: 14.6g Protein: 15.7g

Super Smoothie

Preparation Time: 5 minutes

Cooking Time: 0 minutes

Servings: 4

Ingredients:

- 1 banana, peeled
- 1 cup chopped mango
- 1 cup raspberries
- ¼ cup rolled oats
- 1 carrot, peeled
- 1 cup chopped fresh kale
- 2 tablespoons chopped fresh parsley
- 1 tablespoon flaxseeds
- 1 tablespoon grated fresh ginger
- ½ cup unsweetened soy milk
- 1 cup water

Directions:

1. Put all the ingredients in a food processor, then blitz until glossy and smooth.
2. Serve immediately or chill in the refrigerator for an hour before serving.

Nutrition: Calories: 550 Fat: 39.0g Carbs: 31.0g Fiber: 15.0g Protein: 13.0g

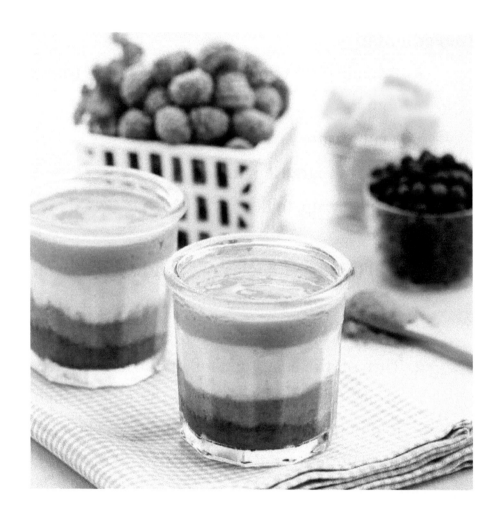

Light Ginger Tea

Preparation Time: 5 minutes

Cooking Time: 10 to 15 minutes

Servings: 2

Ingredients:

- 1 small ginger knob, sliced into four 1-inch chunks
- 4 cups water
- Juice of 1 large lemon
- Maple syrup, to taste

Directions:

1. Add the ginger knob and water in a saucepan, then simmer over medium heat for 10 to 15 minutes.
2. Turn off the heat, then mix in the lemon juice. Strain the liquid to remove the ginger, then fold in the maple syrup and serve.

Nutrition: Calories: 32 Fat: 0.1g Carbs: 8.6g Fiber: 0.1g Protein: 0.1g

Lime and Cucumber Electrolyte Drink

Preparation Time: 5 minutes

Cooking Time: 0 minutes

Servings: 4

Ingredients:

- ¼ cup chopped cucumber
- 1 tablespoon fresh lime juice
- 1 tablespoon apple cider vinegar
- 2 tablespoons maple syrup
- ¼ teaspoon sea salt, optional
- 4 cups water

Directions:

1. Combine all the ingredients in a glass. Stir to mix well.
2. Refrigerate overnight before serving.

Nutrition: Calories: 114 Fat: 0.1g Carbs: 28.9g Fiber: 0.3g Protein: 0.3g

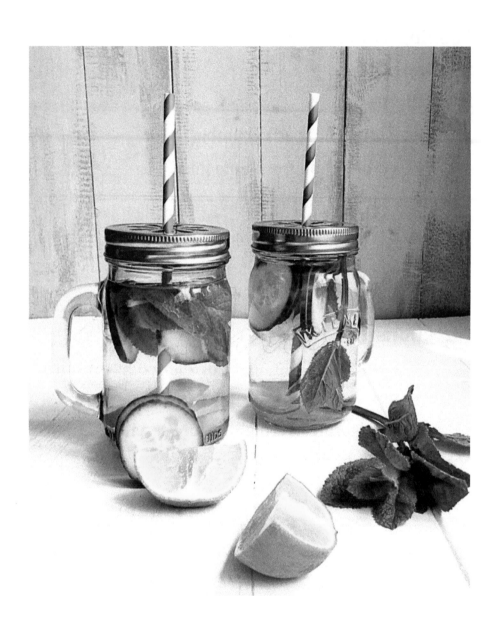

Simple Date Shake

Preparation Time: 10 minutes

Cooking Time: 0 minutes

Servings: 2

Ingredients:

- 5 Medjool dates, pitted, soaked in boiling water for 5 minutes
- ¾ cup unsweetened coconut milk
- 1 teaspoon vanilla extract
- ½ teaspoon fresh lemon juice
- ¼ teaspoon sea salt, optional
- 1½ cups ice

Directions:

1. Put all the ingredients in a food processor, then blitz until it has a milkshake and smooth texture.
2. Serve immediately.

Nutrition: Calories: 380 Fat: 21.6g Carbs: 50.3g Fiber: 6.0g Protein: 3.2g

Beet and Clementine Protein Smoothie

Preparation Time: 10 minutes

Cooking Time: 0 minutes

Servings: 3

Ingredients:

- 1 small beet, peeled and chopped
- 1 clementine, peeled and broken into segments
- ½ ripe banana
- ½ cup raspberries
- 1 tablespoon chia seeds
- 2 tablespoons almond butter
- ¼ teaspoon vanilla extract
- 1 cup unsweetened almond milk
- 1/8 teaspoon fine sea salt, optional

Directions:

1. Combine all the ingredients in a food processor, then pulse on high for 2 minutes or until glossy and creamy.
2. Refrigerate for an hour and serve chilled.

Nutrition: Calories: 526 Fat: 25.4g Carbs: 61.9g Fiber: 17.3g Protein: 20.6g

Matcha Limeade

Preparation Time: 10 minutes

Cooking Time: 0 minutes

Servings: 4

Ingredients:

- 2 tablespoons matcha powder
- ¼ cup raw agave syrup
- 3 cups water, divided
- 1 cup fresh lime juice
- 3 tablespoons chia seeds

Directions:

1. Lightly simmer the matcha, agave syrup, and 1 cup of water in a saucepan over medium heat. Keep stirring until no matcha lumps.
2. Pour the matcha mixture in a large glass, then add the remaining ingredients and stir to mix well.
3. Refrigerate for at least an hour before serving.

Nutrition: Calories: 152 Fat: 4.5g Carbs: 26.8g Fiber: 5.3g Protein: 3.7g

BREAD

Delicious Cheese Bread

Preparation Time: 10 Minutes

Cooking Time: 35 Minutes

Servings: 12

Ingredients:

- Eggs – 2
- All-purpose flour – 2 cups
- Butter – 1/2 cup, melted
- Buttermilk – 1 cup
- Baking soda – 1/2 teaspoon.
- Baking powder – 1/2 teaspoon.
- Sugar – 1 teaspoon.
- Cheddar cheese – 1 cup, shredded
- Salt– 1/2 teaspoon.

Directions:

1. Preheat the oven for 350 F. In a large mixing bowl, mix flour, baking soda, baking powder, sugar, cheese, pepper, and salt.
2. In a small bowl, beat eggs with buttermilk, and butter. Add egg mixture to the flour mixture and mix well.

3. Transfer mixture into the greased 9*5-inch loaf pan and bake in preheated oven for 35-40 minutes.

4. Allow to cool for 15 minutes. Slice and serve.

Nutrition: Calories 202, Carbs 17.6g, Fat 11.9g, Protein 6.2g

Strawberry Bread

Preparation Time: 15 Minutes

Cooking Time: 60 Minutes

Servings: 10

Ingredients:

- Eggs – 2
- All-purpose flour – 2 cups
- Vanilla – 1 teaspoon.
- Vegetable oil – 1/2 cup
- Baking soda – 1 teaspoon.
- Cinnamon – 1/2 teaspoon.
- Brown sugar – 1/2 cup
- White sugar – 1/2 cup
- Fresh strawberries – 2 1/4 cups, chopped
- Salt – 1/2 teaspoon.

Directions:

1. Preheat the oven to 350 F. Grease 9.5-inch loaf pan and set aside.
2. In a mixing bowl, mix together flour, baking soda, cinnamon, brown sugar, white sugar, and salt.

3. In a separate bowl, beat eggs, vanilla, and oil. Stir in strawberries.

4. Add flour mixture to the egg mixture and stir until well combined.

5. Pour batter into the prepared loaf pan and bake in preheated oven for 50-60 minutes.

6. Allow to cool for 10-15 minutes. Slice and serve.

Nutrition: Calories 364, Carbs 40.1g, Fat 21.g, Protein 4.2g

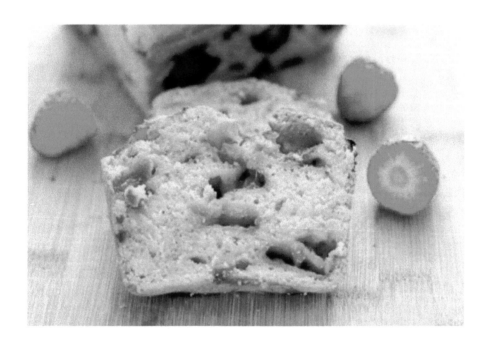

Almond Bread

Preparation Time: 10 Minutes

Cooking Time: 30 Minutes

Servings: 20

Ingredients:

- Eggs – 6, separated
- Cream of tartar – 1/4 teaspoon.
- Baking powder – 3 teaspoon.
- Butter – 4 tablespoons, melted
- Almond flour – 1 1/2 cups
- Salt – 1/4 teaspoon.

Directions:

1. Preheat the oven to 375 F. Grease 8*4-inch loaf pan with butter and set aside. Add egg whites and cream of tartar in a large bowl and beat until soft peaks form.

2. Add almond flour, baking powder, egg yolks, butter, and salt in a food processor and process until combined.

3. Add 1/3 of egg white mixture into the almond flour mixture and process until combined.

Now add remaining egg white mixture and process gently to combine.

4. Pour batter into the prepared loaf pan and bake for 30 minutes. Slice and serve.

Nutrition: Calories 52, Carbs 1g, Fat 4g, Protein 2g

Sweet Rolls

Preparation Time: 2 hours

Cooking Time: 30 Minutes

Servings: 8

Ingredients:

- 2 tablespoons cane sugar
- 1 teaspoon rapid dry yeast
- 2 1/2 tablespoons warm water
- 1/2 cup pineapple juice, plus more for brushing tops of rolls
- 2 tablespoons coconut oil, melted
- 1 3/4 cups unbleached all-purpose flour, plus more for rolling out the dough

Directions:

1. In a small bowl, combine the sugar, yeast, and warm water. Stir gently and set aside for 10 minutes.
2. In another small bowl, combine 1/2 cup of pineapple juice and the coconut oil and stir.
3. Add the yeast mixture to the pineapple mixture and stir gently.

4. Add 1 3/4 cups of flour and mix with your hands until well combined. The dough should not be too sticky. Knead in the bowl for 10 minutes, or until the dough is soft and smooth.

5. Place the dough in an oiled bowl, cover with a clean, damp towel, and place in a warm area for 1 hour to allow it to rise.

6. On a lightly floured surface, knead the dough, incorporating the flour from the surface. Break the dough into 8 equal pieces and form rolls.

7. Place the rolls on an oiled baking pan and allow to rise again for 30 to 40 minutes. Twenty minutes into this second rise, preheat the oven to 375-degree F.

8. Use a pastry brush to brush the tops of the rolls with pineapple juice.

9. Bake for 25 to 30 minutes or until golden brown.

Nutrition: Calories 115, Carbs 2.5g, Fat 11.5g, Protein 6.7g

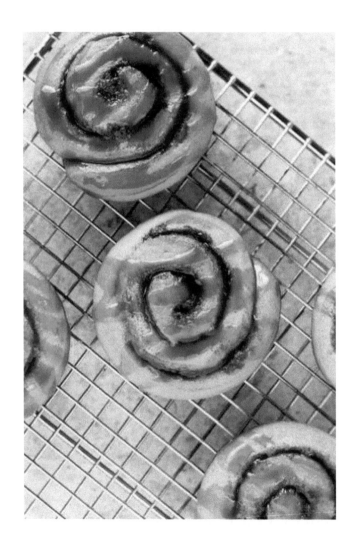

Zero-Fat Carrot Pineapple Loaf

Preparation Time: 20 minutes

Cooking Time: 1.5 hours

Serving Size: 1 ounce (28.3g)

Ingredients:

- 2 ½ cups all-purpose flour
- ¾ cup of sugar
- ½ cup pineapples, crushed
- ½ cup carrots, grated
- ½ cup raisins
- Two teaspoons baking powder
- ½ teaspoon ground cinnamon
- ½ teaspoon salt
- ¼ teaspoon allspice
- ¼ teaspoon nutmeg
- ½ cup applesauce
- One tablespoon molasses

Directions:

1. Put first the wet ingredients into the bread pan before the dry ingredients.
2. Press the "Quick" or "Cake" mode of your bread machine.

3. Allow the machine to complete all cycles.

4. Take out the pan from the machine but wait for another 10 minutes before transferring the bread into a wire rack.

5. Cooldown the bread before slicing.

Nutrition: Calories: 70 | Carbohydrates: 16g Fat: 0g | Protein: 1g

Autumn Treasures Loaf

Preparation Time: 15 minutes

Cooking Time: 1/5 hours

Serving Size: 1 ounce (28.3g)

Ingredients:

- 1 cup all-purpose flour
- ½ cup dried fruit, chopped
- ¼ cup pecans, chopped
- ¼ cup of sugar
- Two tablespoons baking powder
- One teaspoon salt
- ¼ teaspoon of baking soda
- ½ teaspoon ground nutmeg
- 1 cup apple juice
- ¼ cup of vegetable oil
- Three tablespoons aquafaba
- One teaspoon of vanilla extract

Directions:

1. Add all wet ingredients first to the bread pan before the dry ingredients.
2. Turn on the bread machine with the "Quick" or "Cake" setting.

3. Wait for all cycles to be finished.

4. Remove the bread pan from the machine.

5. After 10 minutes, transfer the bread from the pan into a wire rack.

6. Slice the bread only when it has completely cooled down.

Nutrition: Calories: 80 | Carbohydrates: 12g Fat: 3g | Protein: 1g

Beer Bread

Preparation Time: 10-15 minutes

Cooking Time: 2.5-3 hours

Serving Size: 2 ounces (56.7g)

Ingredients:

- 3 cups bread flour
- Two tablespoons sugar
- Two ¼ teaspoons yeast
- 1 ½ teaspoons salt
- 2/3 cup beer
- 1/3 cup water
- Two tablespoons vegetable oil

Directions:

1. Add all ingredients into a pan in this order: water, beer, oil, salt, sugar, flour, and yeast.
2. Start the bread machine with the "Basic" or "Normal" mode on and light to medium crust colour.
3. Let the machine complete all cycles.
4. Take out the pan from the machine.
5. Transfer the beer bread into a wire rack to cool it down for about an hour.

6. Cut into 12 slices and serve.

Nutrition: Calories: 130 | Carbohydrates: 25g Fat: 1g | Protein: 4g

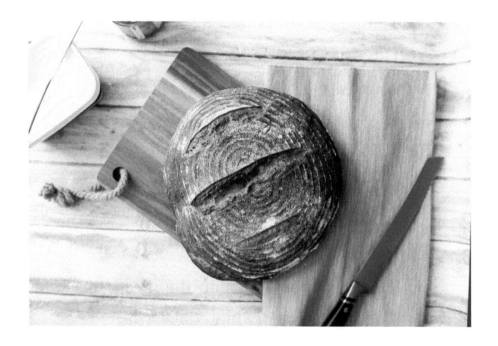

Onion and Mushroom Bread

Preparation Time: 10 minutes

Cooking Time: 1 hour

Serving Size: 2 ounces (56.7g)

Ingredients:

- 4 ounces mushrooms, chopped
- 4 cups bread flour
- Three tablespoons sugar
- Four teaspoons fast-acting yeast
- Four teaspoons dried onions, minced
- 1 ½ teaspoons salt
- ½ teaspoon garlic powder
- ¾ cup of water

Directions:

1. Pour the water first into the bread pan, and then add all the dry ingredients.
2. Press the "Fast" cycle mode of the bread machine.
3. Wait until all cycles are completed.
4. Transfer the bread from the pan into a wire rack.

5. Wait for one hour before slicing the bread into 12 pieces.

6. Serving Size: 2 ounces per slice

Nutrition: Calories: 120 | Carbohydrates: 25g Fat: 0g | Protein: 5g

Low-Carb Multigrain Bread

Preparation Time: 15 minutes

Cooking Time: 1.5 hours

Serving Size: 1 ounce (28.3g)

Ingredients:

- ¾ cup whole-wheat flour
- ¼ cup cornmeal
- ¼ cup oatmeal
- Two tablespoons 7-grain cereals
- Two tablespoons baking powder
- One teaspoon salt
- ¼ teaspoon baking soda
- ¾ cup of water
- ¼ cup of vegetable oil
- ¼ cup of orange juice
- Three tablespoons aquafaba

Directions:

1. In the bread pan, add the wet ingredients first, then the dry ingredients.
2. Press the "Quick" or "Cake" mode of your bread machine.
3. Wait until all cycles are through.

4. Remove the bread pan from the machine.

5. Let the bread rest for 10 minutes in the pan before taking it out to cool down further.

6. Slice the bread after an hour has passed.

Nutrition: Calories: 60 | Carbohydrates: 9g Fat: 2g | Protein: 1g

Mashed Potato Bread

Preparation Time: 40 minutes

Cooking Time: 2.5-3 hours

Serving Size: 2 ounces (56.7g) per slice

Ingredients:

- 2 1/3 cups bread flour
- ½ cup mashed potatoes
- One tablespoon sugar
- 1 ½ teaspoons yeast
- ¾ teaspoon salt
- ¼ cup potato water
- One tablespoon ground flax seeds
- Four teaspoons oil

Directions:

1. Put the ingredients into the pan in this order: potato water, oil, flax seeds, mashed potatoes, sugar, salt, flour, and yeast.
2. Ready the bread machine by pressing the "Basic" or "Normal" mode with a medium crust colour setting.
3. Allow the bread machine to finish all cycles.
4. Remove the bread pan from the machine.

5. Carefully take the bread from the pan.

6. Put the bread on a wire rack, then cool down before slicing.

Nutrition: Calories: 140 Carbohydrates: 26 g

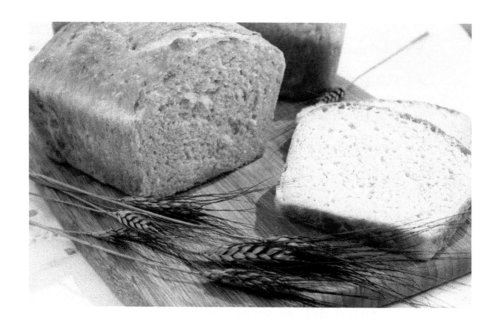

Healthy Celery Loaf

Preparation Time: 2 hours 40 minutes

Cooking Time: 50 minutes

Servings: 1 loaf

Ingredients:

- 1 can (10 ounces) cream of celery soup
- tablespoons coconut milk, heated
- 1 tablespoon vegetable oil
- 1¼ teaspoons celery salt
- ¾ cup celery, fresh/sliced thin
- 1 tablespoon celery leaves, fresh, chopped
- 1 whole egg
- ¼ teaspoon sugar
- cups bread flour
- ¼ teaspoon ginger
- ½ cup quick-cooking oats
- tablespoons gluten
- teaspoons celery seeds
- 1 pack of active dry yeast

Directions:

1 Add all the ingredients to your bread machine, carefully following the instructions of the manufacturer

2 Set the program of your bread machine to Basic/White Bread and set crust type to Medium

3 Press START

4 Wait until the cycle completes

5 Once the loaf is ready, take the bucket out and let the loaf cool for 5 minutes

6 Gently shake the bucket to remove the loaf

7 Transfer to a cooling rack, slice and serve

8 Enjoy!

Nutrition: Calories: 73 Cal Fat: 4 g Carbohydrates: 8 g Protein: 3 g Fiber: 1 g

Broccoli and Cauliflower Bread

Preparation Time: 2 hours 20 minutes

Cooking Time: 50 minutes

Servings: 1 loaf

Ingredients:

- ¼ cup water
- tablespoons olive oil
- 1 egg white
- 1 teaspoon lemon juice
- 2/3 cup grated cheddar cheese
- tablespoons green onion
- ½ cup broccoli, chopped
- ½ cup cauliflower, chopped
- ½ teaspoon lemon pepper seasoning
- cups bread flour
- 1 teaspoon bread machine yeast

Directions:

1 Add all of the ingredients to your bread machine, carefully following the instructions of the manufacturer

2 Set the program of your bread machine to Basic/White Bread and set crust type to Medium

3 Press START

4 Wait until the cycle completes

5 Once the loaf is ready, take the bucket out and let the loaf cool for 5 minutes

6 Gently shake the bucket to remove the loaf

7 Transfer to a cooling rack, slice and serve

8 Enjoy!

Nutrition: Calories: 156 Cal Fat: 8 g Carbohydrates: 17 g Protein: 5 g Fiber: 2 g

Potato Bread

Preparation Time: 3 hours

Cooking Time: 45 minutes

Servings: 2 loaves

Ingredients:

- 1 3/4 teaspoon active dry yeast
- tablespoon dry milk
- 1/4 cup instant potato flakes
- tablespoon sugar
- cups bread flour
- 1 1/4 teaspoon salt
- tablespoon butter
- 1 3/8 cups water

Directions:

1 Put all the liquid ingredients in the pan. Add all the dry ingredients, except the yeast. Form a shallow hole in the middle of the dry ingredients and place the yeast.

2 Secure the pan in the machine and close the lid. Choose the basic setting and your desired color of the crust. Press starts.

3 Allow the bread to cool before slicing.

Nutrition: Calories: 35calories; Total Carbohydrate: 19 g Total Fat: 0 g Protein: 4 g

Onion Potato Bread

Preparation Time: 1 hour 20 minutes

Cooking Time: 45 minutes

Servings: 2 loaves

Ingredients:

- tablespoon quick rise yeast
- cups bread flour
- 1 1/2 teaspoon seasoned salt
- tablespoon sugar
- 2/3 cup baked potatoes, mashed
- 1 1/2 cup onions, minced
- large eggs
- tablespoon oil
- 3/4 cup hot water, with the temperature of 115 to 125 degrees F (46 to 51 degrees C)

Directions:

1 Put the liquid ingredients in the pan. Add the dry ingredients, except the yeast. Form a shallow well in the middle using your hand and put the yeast.

2 Place the pan in the machine, close the lid and turn it on. Select the express bake 80 setting and start the machine.

3 Once the bread is cooked, leave on a wire rack for 20 minutes or until cooled.

Nutrition: Calories: 160calories; Total Carbohydrate: 44 g Total Fat: 2 g Protein: 6 g

Spinach Bread

Preparation Time: 2 hours 20 minutes

Cooking Time: 40 minutes

Servings: 1 loaf

Ingredients:

- 1 cup water
- 1 tablespoon vegetable oil
- 1/2 cup frozen chopped spinach, thawed and drained
- cups all-purpose flour
- 1/2 cup shredded Cheddar cheese
- 1 teaspoon salt
- 1 tablespoon white sugar
- 1/2 teaspoon ground black pepper
- 1/2 teaspoons active dry yeast

Directions:

1   In the pan of bread machine, put all ingredients according to the suggested order of manufacture. Set white bread cycle.

Nutrition: Calories: 121 calories; Total Carbohydrate: 20.5 g Cholesterol: 4 mg Total Fat: 2.5 g Protein: 4 g Sodium: 184 mg

Curd Bread

Preparation Time: 4 hours

Cooking Time: 15 minutes

Servings: 12

Ingredients:

- ¾ cup lukewarm water
- 2/3 cups wheat bread machine flour
- ¾ cup cottage cheese
- Tablespoon softened butter
- Tablespoon white sugar
- 1½ teaspoon sea salt
- 1½ Tablespoon sesame seeds
- Tablespoon dried onions
- 1¼ teaspoon bread machine yeast

Directions:

1. Place all the dry and liquid ingredients in the pan and follow the instructions for your bread machine.

2. Pay particular attention to measuring the ingredients. Use a measuring cup, measuring spoon, and kitchen scales to do so.

3. Set the baking program to BASIC and the crust type to MEDIUM.

4. If the dough is too dense or too wet, adjust the amount of flour and liquid in the recipe.

5. When the program has ended, take the pan out of the bread machine and let cool for 5 minutes.

6. Shake the loaf out of the pan. If necessary, use a spatula.

7. Wrap the bread with a kitchen towel and set it aside for an hour. Otherwise, you can cool it on a wire rack.

Nutrition: Calories: 277 calories; Total Carbohydrate: 48.4 g Cholesterol: 9 g Total Fat: 4.7g Protein: 9.4 g Sodium: 547 mg Sugar: 3.3 g

Curvy Carrot Bread

Preparation Time: 2 hours

Cooking Time: 15 minutes

Servings: 12

Ingredients:

- ¾ cup milk, lukewarm
- tablespoons butter, melted at room temperature
- 1 tablespoon honey
- ¾ teaspoon ground nutmeg
- ½ teaspoon salt
- 1 ½ cups shredded carrot
- cups white bread flour
- ¼ teaspoons bread machine or active dry yeast

Directions:

1 Take 1 ½ pound size loaf pan and first add the liquid ingredients and then add the dry ingredients.

2 Place the loaf pan in the machine and close its top lid.

3 Plug the bread machine into power socket. For selecting a bread cycle, press "Quick Bread/Rapid

Bread" and for selecting a crust type, press "Light" or "Medium".

4 Start the machine and it will start preparing the bread.

5 After the bread loaf is completed, open the lid and take out the loaf pan.

6 Allow the pan to cool down for 10-15 minutes on a wire rack. Gently shake the pan and remove the bread loaf.

7 Make slices and serve.

Nutrition: Calories: 142 calories; Total Carbohydrate: 32.2 g Cholesterol: 0 g Total Fat: 0.8 g Protein: 2.33 g

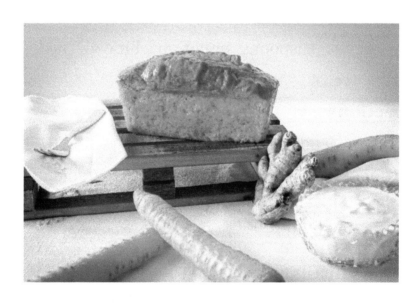

Potato Rosemary Bread

Preparation Time: 3 hours

Cooking Time: 30 minutes

Servings: 20

Ingredients:

- cups bread flour, sifted
- 1 tablespoon white sugar
- 1 tablespoon sunflower oil
- 1½ teaspoons salt
- 1½ cups lukewarm water
- 1 teaspoon active dry yeast
- 1 cup potatoes, mashed
- teaspoons crushed rosemary

Directions:

1 Prepare all the ingredients for your bread and measuring means (a cup, a spoon, kitchen scales).

2 Carefully measure the ingredients into the pan, except the potato and rosemary.

3 Place all the ingredients into the bread bucket in the right order, following the manual for your bread machine.

4 Close the cover.

5 Select the program of your bread machine to BREAD with FILLINGS and choose the crust color to MEDIUM.

6 Press START.

7 After the signal, put the mashed potato and rosemary to the dough.

8 Wait until the program completes.

9 When done, take the bucket out and let it cool for 5-10 minutes.

10 Shake the loaf from the pan and let cool for 30 minutes on a cooling rack.

11 Slice, serve and enjoy the taste of fragrant homemade bread.

Nutrition: Calories: 106 calories; Total Carbohydrate: 21 g Total Fat: 1 g Protein: 2.9 g Sodium: 641 mg Fiber: 1 g Sugar: 0.8 g

Beetroot Prune Bread

Preparation Time: 3 hours

Cooking Time: 30 minutes

Servings: 20

Ingredients:

- 1½ cups lukewarm beet broth
- 5¼ cups all-purpose flour
- 1 cup beet puree
- 1 cup prunes, chopped
- tablespoons extra virgin olive oil
- tablespoons dry cream
- 1 tablespoon brown sugar
- teaspoons active dry yeast
- 1 tablespoon whole milk
- teaspoons sea salt

Directions:

1 Prepare all the ingredients for your bread and measuring means (a cup, a spoon, kitchen scales).

2 Carefully measure the ingredients into the pan, except the prunes.

3 Place all the ingredients into the bread bucket in the right order, following the manual for your bread machine.

4 Close the cover.

5 Select the program of your bread machine to BASIC and choose the crust color to MEDIUM.

6 Press START.

7 After the signal, put the prunes to the dough.

8 Wait until the program completes.

9 When done, take the bucket out and let it cool for 5-10 minutes.

10 Shake the loaf from the pan and let cool for 30 minutes on a cooling rack.

11 Slice, serve and enjoy the taste of fragrant homemade bread.

Nutrition: Calories: 443 calories; Total Carbohydrate: 81.1 g Total Fat: 8.2 g Protein: 9.9 g Sodium: 604 mg Fiber: 4.4 g Sugar: 11.7 g

SAUCES, DRESSINGS, AND DIPS

Satay Sauce

Preparation Time: 5 minutes

Cooking Time: 8 minutes

Servings: 2

Ingredients:

- ½ yellow onion, diced
- 3 garlic cloves, minced
- 1 fresh red chile, thinly sliced (optional)
- 1-inch (2.5-cm) piece fresh ginger, peeled and minced
- ¼ cup smooth peanut butter
- 2 tablespoons coconut aminos
- 1 (13.5-ounce / 383-g) can unsweetened coconut milk
- ¼ teaspoon freshly ground black pepper
- ¼ teaspoon salt (optional)

Directions:

1. Heat a large nonstick skillet over medium-high heat until hot.
2. Add the onion, garlic cloves, chile (if desired), and ginger to the skillet, and sauté for 2 minutes.

3. Pour in the peanut butter and coconut aminos and stir well. Add the coconut milk, black pepper, and salt (if desired) and continue whisking, or until the sauce is just beginning to bubble and thicken.

4. Remove the sauce from the heat to a bowl. Taste and adjust the seasoning if necessary.

Nutrition: Calories: 322 Fat: 28.8g Carbs: 9.4gProtein: 6.3gFiber: 1.8g

Tahini BBQ Sauce

Preparation Time: 10 minutes

Cooking Time: 0 minutes

Servings: 4

Ingredients:

- ½ cup water
- ¼ cup red miso
- 3 cloves garlic, minced
- 1-inch (2.5 cm) piece ginger, peeled and minced
- 2 tablespoons rice vinegar
- 2 tablespoons tahini
- 2 tablespoons chili paste or chili sauce
- 1 tablespoon date sugar
- ½ teaspoon crushed red pepper (optional)

Directions:

1. Place all the ingredients in a food processor, and purée until thoroughly mixed and smooth. You can thin the sauce out by stirring in ½ cup of water or keep it thick.

2. Transfer to the refrigerator to chill until ready to serve.

Nutrition: Calories: 206 Fat: 10.2g Carbs: 21.3g Protein: 7.2g Fiber: 4.4g

Homemade Tzatziki Sauce

Preparation Time: 20 minutes

Cooking Time: 0 minutes

Servings: 1

Ingredients:

- 2 ounces (57 g) raw, unsalted cashews (about ½ cup)
- 2 tablespoons lemon juice
- 1/3 cup water
- 1 small clove garlic
- 1 cup chopped cucumber, peeled
- 2 tablespoons fresh dill

Directions:

1. In a blender, add the cashews, lemon juice, water, and garlic. Keep it aside for at least 15 minutes to soften the cashews.

2. Blend the ingredients until smooth. Stir in the chopped cucumber and dill and continue to blend until it reaches your desired consistency. It doesn't need to be totally smooth. Feel free to add more water if you like a thinner consistency.

3. Transfer to an airtight container and chill for at least 30 minutes for best flavors.

4. Bring the sauce to room temperature and shake well before serving.

Nutrition: Calories: 208 Fat: 13.5g Carbs: 15.0 g Protein: 6.7g Fiber: 2.8g

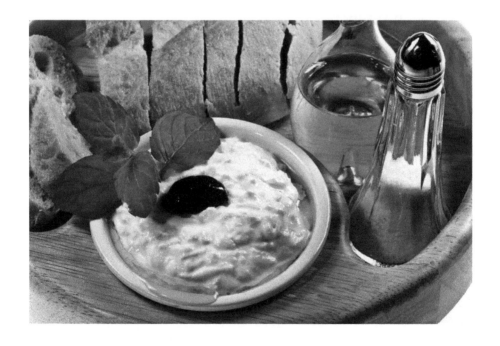

Avocado-dill Dressing

Preparation Time: 20 minutes

Cooking Time: 0 minutes

Servings: 1

Ingredients:

- 2 ounces (57 g) raw, unsalted cashews (about ½ cup)
- ½ cup water
- 3 tablespoons lemon juice
- ½ medium, ripe avocado, chopped
- 1 medium clove garlic
- 2 tablespoons chopped fresh dill
- 2 green onions, white and green parts, chopped

Directions:

1. Put the cashews, water, lemon juice, avocado, and garlic into a blender. Keep it aside for at least 15 minutes to soften the cashews.
2. Blend until everything is fully mixed. Fold in the dill and green onions, and blend briefly to retain some texture.

3. Store in an airtight container in the fridge for up to 3 days and stir well before serving.

Nutrition: Calories: 312 Fat: 21.1g Carbs: 22.6g Protein: 8.0g Fiber: 7.1g

Easy Lemon Tahini Dressing

Preparation Time: 5 minutes

Cooking Time: 0 minutes

Servings: 1

Ingredients:

- ½ cup tahini
- ¼ cup fresh lemon juice (about 2 lemons)
- 1 teaspoon maple syrup
- 1 small garlic clove, chopped
- 1/8 teaspoon black pepper
- ¼ teaspoon salt (optional)
- ¼ to ½ cup water

Directions:

1. Process the tahini, lemon juice, maple syrup, garlic, black pepper, and salt (if desired) in a blender (high-speed blenders work best for this). Gradually add the water until the mixture is completely smooth.
2. Store in an airtight container in the fridge for up to 5 days.

Nutrition: Calories: 128 Fat: 9.6g Carbs: 6.8g Protein: 3.6g Fiber: 1.9g

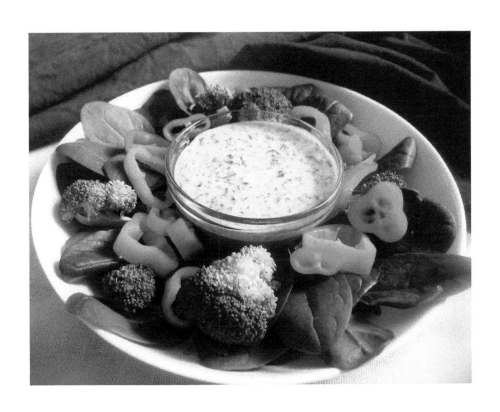

Sweet Mango and Orange Dressing

Preparation Time: 5 minutes

Cooking Time: 0 minutes

Servings: 1

Ingredients:

- 1 cup (165 g) diced mango, thawed if frozen
- ½ cup orange juice
- 2 tablespoons rice vinegar
- 2 tablespoons fresh lime juice
- ¼ teaspoon salt (optional)
- 1 teaspoon date sugar (optional)
- 2 tablespoons chopped cilantro

Directions:

1. Pulse all the ingredients except for the cilantro in a food processor until it reaches the consistency you like. Add the cilantro and whisk well.
2. Store in an airtight container in the fridge for up to 2 days.

Nutrition: Calories: 32 Fat: 0.1g Carbs: 7.4g Protein: 0.3g Fiber: 0.5g

SALADS

Cashew Siam Salad

Preparation Time: 10 minutes

Cooking Time: 3 minutes

Servings: 4

Ingredients:

Salad:

- 4 cups baby spinach, rinsed, drained
- ½ cup pickled red cabbage

Dressing:

- 1-inch piece ginger, finely chopped
- 1 tsp. chili garlic paste
- 1 tbsp. soy sauce
- ½ tbsp. rice vinegar
- 1 tbsp. sesame oil
- 3 tbsp. avocado oil

Toppings:

- ½ cup raw cashews, unsalted
- ¼ cup fresh cilantro, chopped

Directions:

1. Put the spinach and red cabbage in a large bowl. Toss to combine and set the salad aside.

2. Toast the cashews in a frying pan over medium-high heat, stirring occasionally until the cashews are golden brown. This should take about 3 minutes. Turn off the heat and set the frying pan aside.

3. Mix all the dressing ingredients in medium-sized bowl and use a spoon to mix them into a smooth dressing.

4. Pour the dressing over the spinach salad and top with the toasted cashews.

5. Toss the salad to combine all ingredients and transfer the large bowl to the fridge. Allow the salad to chill for up to one hour – doing so will guarantee a better flavor. Alternatively, the salad can be served right away, topped with the optional cilantro. Enjoy!

Nutrition: Calories 160 Total Fat 12.9g Saturated Fat 2.4g Cholesterol 0mg Sodium 265mg Total Carbohydrate 9.1g Dietary Fiber 2.1g Total Sugars 1.4g Protein 4.1g Vitamin D 0mcg Calcium 45mg Iron 2mg Potassium 344mg

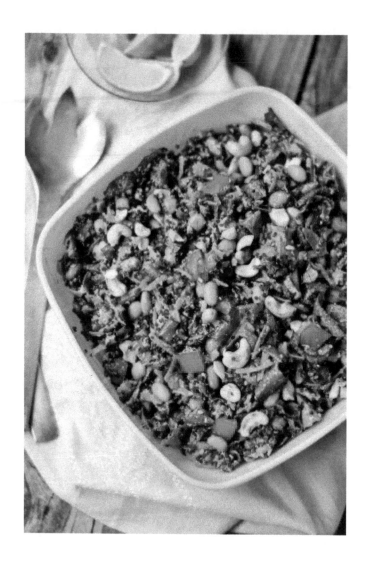

Cucumber Edamame Salad

Preparation Time: 5 minutes

Cooking Time: 8 minutes

Servings: 2

Ingredients:

- 3 tbsp. avocado oil
- 1 cup cucumber, sliced into thin rounds
- ½ cup fresh sugar snap peas, sliced or whole
- ½ cup fresh edamame
- ¼ cup radish, sliced
- 1 large Hass avocado, peeled, pitted, sliced
- 1 nori sheet, crumbled
- 2 tsp. roasted sesame seeds
- 1 tsp. salt

Directions:

1. Bring a medium-sized pot filled halfway with water to a boil over medium-high heat.
2. Add the sugar snaps and cook them for about 2 minutes.
3. Take the pot off the heat, drain the excess water, transfer the sugar snaps to a medium-sized bowl and set aside for now.

4. Fill the pot with water again, add the teaspoon of salt and bring to a boil over medium-high heat.

5. Add the edamame to the pot and let them cook for about 6 minutes.

6. Take the pot off the heat, drain the excess water, transfer the soybeans to the bowl with sugar snaps and let them cool down for about 5 minutes.

7. Combine all ingredients, except the nori crumbs and roasted sesame seeds, in a medium-sized bowl.

8. Carefully stir, using a spoon, until all ingredients are evenly coated in oil.

9. Top the salad with the nori crumbs and roasted sesame seeds.

10. Transfer the bowl to the fridge and allow the salad to cool for at least 30 minutes.

11. Serve chilled and enjoy!

Nutrition: Calories 182 Total Fat 10.9g Saturated Fat 1.3g Cholesterol 0mg Sodium 1182mg Total Carbohydrate 14.2g Dietary Fiber 5.4g Total Sugars 1.9g

Protein 10.7g Vitamin D 0mcg, Calcium 181mg Iron 4mg Potassium 619mg

Lentil, Lemon & Mushroom Salad

Preparation Time: 10 minutes

Cooking Time: 0 minutes

Servings: 2

Ingredients:

- ½ cup dry lentils of choice
- 2 cups vegetable broth
- 3 cups mushrooms, thickly sliced
- 1 cup sweet or purple onion, chopped
- 4 tsp. extra virgin olive oil
- 2 tbsp. garlic powder
- ¼ tsp. chili flakes
- 1 tbsp. lemon juice
- 2 tbsp. cilantro, chopped
- ½ cup arugula
- ¼ tsp Salt
- ¼ tsp pepper

Directions:

1. Sprout the lentils according the method. (Don't cook them).
2. Place the vegetable stock in a deep saucepan and bring it to a boil.

3. Add the lentils to the boiling broth, cover the pan, and cook for about 5 minutes over low heat until the lentils are a bit tender.

4. Remove the pan from heat and drain the excess water.

5. Put a frying pan over high heat and add 2 tablespoons of olive oil.

6. Add the onions, garlic, and chili flakes, and cook until the onions are almost translucent, around 5 to 10 minutes while stirring.

7. Add the mushrooms to the frying pan and mix in thoroughly. Continue cooking until the onions are completely translucent and the mushrooms have softened; remove the pan from the heat.

8. Mix the lentils, onions, mushrooms, and garlic in a large bowl.

9. Add the lemon juice and the remaining olive oil. Toss or stir to combine everything thoroughly.

10. Serve the mushroom/onion mixture over some arugala in bowl, adding salt and pepper to taste, or store and enjoy later!

Nutrition: Calories 365 Total Fat 11.7g Saturated Fat 1.9g Cholesterol 0mg Sodium 1071mg Total Carbohydrate 45.2g Dietary Fiber 18g Total Sugars 8.2g Protein 22.8g Vitamin D 378mcg Calcium 67mg Iron 8mg Potassium 1212mg

Sweet Potato & Black Bean Protein Salad

Preparation Time: 15 minutes

Cooking Time: 0 minutes

Servings: 2

Ingredients:

- 1 cup dry black beans
- 4 cups of spinach
- 1 medium sweet potato
- 1 cup purple onion, chopped
- 2 tbsp. olive oil
- 2 tbsp. lime juice
- 1 tbsp. minced garlic
- ½ tbsp. chili powder
- ¼ tsp. cayenne
- ¼ cup parsley
- ¼ tsp Salt
- ¼ tsp pepper

Directions:

1. Prepare the black beans according to the method.
2. Preheat the oven to 400°F.

3. Cut the sweet potato into ¼-inch cubes and put these in a medium-sized bowl. Add the onions, 1 tablespoon of olive oil, and salt to taste.

4. Toss the ingredients until the sweet potatoes and onions are completely coated.

5. Transfer the ingredients to a baking sheet lined with parchment paper and spread them out in a single layer.

6. Put the baking sheet in the oven and roast until the sweet potatoes are starting to turn brown and crispy, around 40 minutes.

7. Meanwhile, combine the remaining olive oil, lime juice, garlic, chili powder, and cayenne thoroughly in a large bowl, until no lumps remain.

8. Remove the sweet potatoes and onions from the oven and transfer them to the large bowl.

9. Add the cooked black beans, parsley, and a pinch of salt.

10. Toss everything until well combined.

11. Then mix in the spinach and serve in desired portions with additional salt and pepper.

12. Store or enjoy!

Nutrition: Calories 558 Total Fat 16.2g Saturated Fat 2.5g Cholesterol 0mg Sodium 390mg Total Carbohydrate 84g Dietary Fiber 20.4g Total Sugars 8.9g Protein 25.3g Vitamin D 0mcg Calcium 220mg Iron 10mg Potassium 2243mg

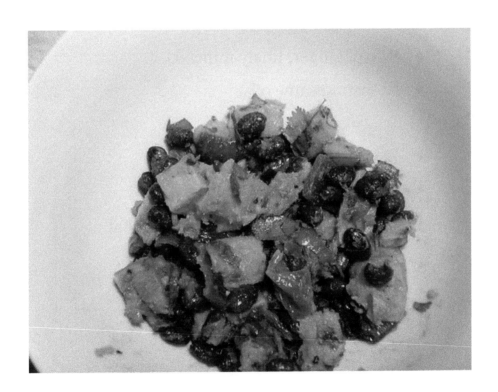

Edamame & Ginger Citrus Salad

Preparation Time: 15 minutes

Cooking Time: 0 minutes

Servings: 3

Ingredients:

Dressing:

- ¼ cup orange juice
- 1 tsp. lime juice
- ½ tbsp. maple syrup
- ½ tsp. ginger, finely minced
- ½ tbsp. sesame oil

Salad:

- ½ cup dry green lentils
- 2 cups carrots, shredded
- 4 cups kale, fresh or frozen, chopped
- 1 cup edamame, shelled
- 1 tablespoon roasted sesame seeds
- 2 tsp. mint, chopped
- Salt and pepper to taste
- 1 small avocado, peeled, pitted, diced

Directions:

1. Prepare the lentils according to the method.

2. Combine the orange and lime juices, maple syrup, and ginger in a small bowl. Mix with a whisk while slowly adding the sesame oil.

3. Add the cooked lentils, carrots, kale, edamame, sesame seeds, and mint to a large bowl.

4. Add the dressing and stir well until all the ingredients are coated evenly.

5. Store or serve topped with avocado and an additional sprinkle of mint.

Nutrition: Calories 507 Total Fat 23.1g Saturated Fat 4g Cholesterol 0mg Sodium 303mg Total Carbohydrate 56.8g Dietary Fiber 21.6g Total Sugars 8.4g Protein 24.6g Vitamin D 0mcg Calcium 374mg Iron 8mg Potassium 1911mg

Lightning Source UK Ltd.
Milton Keynes UK
UKHW020801110621
385329UK00001B/143